The Fe...

Lose weight, gain health. Recipes and tips for the 5:2 diet.

by

Mags Casey

and

Clive Mingham

Copyright © 2013,

M. A. Casey

and

C. G. Mingham.

All rights reserved.

To Dr Michael Mosley
for his inspiring TV documentary
and to all scientists working to
understand the health
benefits of intermittent calorie
restriction.

Table of Contents

Introduction	5
Breakfasts	10
Lunches	15
Soups	18
Evening Meals	25
Drinks	39
Freebies	40
Snacks	41
Calorie Counter	43
Tips	49
Results	51

Introduction

After 12 weeks on the Feast and Fast Diet we found that it *worked* so we wrote up what we did as an e-book. This physical book is the re-formatted e-book in which recipes occupy either a single page or two facing pages so that you don't need to turn over with grubby fingers as you make them. Space where you can add your own notes has been included where possible.

Our main aim was not to lose weight, although we have steadily lost quite a bit of weight (see the Results section and the cover picture which shows that we need some new clothes!), but to improve our overall health. We both *feel* healthier and we are continuing with the diet which has become even easier to follow as we got used to it.

The original motivation for this diet was that Clive has high cholesterol (probably not helped by his fondness for pies). According to his doctor, Clive's initial readings put him in the Fredrickson Type II B category (not a good thing). His doctor offered to prescribe him Statins which he declined.

We wanted to take control of our own health as far as possible so started researching diets. This was interrupted by three weeks in France during the summer of 2012 when all thoughts of diets were smothered under mounds of cream, croissants and confit of duck. One day Clive ate a whole baked Camembert with a plateful of chips and sliced meats. Something had to change...

When we returned home we watched a TV documentary which presented a compelling argument for the health benefits of intermittent fasting backed up by scientific studies. This gave rise to the 5:2 diet where participants consume a small number of calories on 2 'fasting' days per week and eat normally during the other 5 'feasting' days. It's the feast-fast nature of the diet that gives the health benefits (and weight loss) although we don't pretend to understand how it works (it's something to do with the hormone, IGF-1 for those who are interested). The 5:2 diet has produced some amazing results, some of which are:

- lower cholesterol readings, particularly of 'bad' (LDL) cholesterol
- weight loss
- improved memory
- reduced risk of Alzheimer's
- reduced risk of Parkinson's
- reduced risk of diabetes

Clive decided to follow this diet and Mags went along to be supportive. When we looked for interesting low calorie meals to eat on our 'fasting' days there wasn't much handy information out there. So we decided to put together this simple, easy to follow guide to help us stick to the 2 days out of 7 when we had to eat much less than normal.

We've adopted the following approach on 'fasting' days:

- 500 kcal for women (Mags) and 600 kcal for men (Clive)
- 3 meals a day with about the same number of calories in each meal
- healthy and tasty food
- avoiding additives and nasty chemicals
- getting as much as possible for the calories so we feel like we're eating a proper meal
- easy to find ingredients
- easy to prepare
- don't 'fast' on consecutive days

The following guide to what we eat on our 'fasting' days should give enough ideas to get you through a whole month without having to repeat main meals. To be honest you can eat whatever you like on a 'fasting' day as long as you don't exceed the 500 or 600 kcal daily limit. Research seems to indicate that you can eat what you like on a 'feasting' day but common sense says that you should try to eat healthy food. If you have any medical issues you should get advice from your doctor before starting this diet. Good luck and let us know how you get on by tweeting us at: magsclive

Breakfasts

Do eat breakfast as it will kick start your metabolism and stop you feeling crabby! Try to eat later in the morning as there's some evidence to show that if you delay eating your 'fasting' food for 16 hours after your previous meal this will be beneficial in the overall scheme of things. So, if your previous meal was at 6pm then try to eat your 'fasting' breakfast at 10am. Don't worry if you can't do this (Clive can't) as the diet still works.

My Notes

Porridge

Porridge (i.e. oats and water) is brilliant! It fills you up, is good for you, and releases its energy slowly, so you won't feel hungry an hour later. Porridge is our usual breakfast.

1.5oz (40g) oats = 150 kcal (that's about 4 heaped dessert spoons of oats if you can't be bothered to weigh it out).

Method

Put the oats in a bowl, mix with water (calorie free!) and microwave for 2 mins on medium power. Stir and add more water to bulk it up then microwave for a further 2 mins on medium power. Easy!

You can add things to make the porridge taste better and fill you up more. Because Mags needs fewer calories than Clive, she usually has 1oz (30g) of porridge (110 kcal) and then adds something else for interest e.g.

sliced small banana = 40 kcal

handful of raisins or sultanas = 40 kcal

chopped-up small apple = 40 kcal

teaspoon of honey or syrup = 25 kcal

My Notes

Eggs and Rice Cakes (140 kcal)

1 medium sized egg = 80 kcals

2 rice cakes = 60 kcals

Method

Boil the egg (or scramble with water). You can add salt and pepper but beware butter! Unfortunately you can't cut rice cakes in to soldiers to dip in to your egg so save that for a 'feasting' day.

Smoothies (200 kcal)

Smoothies are quick to make if you have a blender and are a great way of getting some of your 5 a day. Put together a combination of:

small banana = 40 kcal

small tub of low fat yoghurt = 50 kcal

small glass of fruit juice and water = 60 kcal

handful of strawberries, raspberries, blackberries, blueberries = 50 kcal

Toasted Muffin and Topping (150 kcal)

Split and toast an English muffin (or crumpet) = 130 kcal.

Top with a handful of strawberries = 20 kcal.

You can't have butter but you'll get used to it!

Fruit Salad (200 kcal)

Fresh fruit salad is nutritious but not particularly filling. Our usual one is:

1 medium apple
1 medium orange
1 small banana
1.5oz (45ml) low-fat natural yoghurt

My Notes

Lunches

Here are some of our common lunches. Also don't forget raw veg as you can have a lot for not many calories – see the Calorie Counter section and experiment with what you like to eat. Send us your best tips!

Rice Cakes (100 kcal + kcal of topping)

Rice cakes are great and range between 25 and 30 kcal per cake. They are a good substitute for much more calorific bread. So you could have 4 for lunch with a healthy topping. This could easily be taken to work with you without the need for much preparation. Have what you fancy for topping within reason, e.g.

3.5oz (100g) low fat cottage cheese = 60 kcal
half a tin of sardines = 60 kcal
mushroom spread (from health food shops) = 10 kcal per rice cake
a third of a tin of baked beans = 110 kcal

low-fat hummus, thinly spread = 60 kcal

Salads

Mix and match your favorite ingredients using the Calorie Counter at the end of this book. Some of our typical salad combinations are:

mixed seed, chicken and tomato
potato and cumin
mackerel and peas
green leaves and prawn

My Notes

Yummy Avocado, Rocket and Roast Veg Salad (175 kcal)

half an avocado = 115 kcal

handful of roasted tomatoes = 30 kcal

green pepper = 15 kcal

a whole bag of rocket = 15 kcal!

Baked Potatoes

Baked potatoes are quick and easy but you can't have a huge one! A medium potato weighing 7oz (200g) contains around 165 kcal and takes about 10 minutes to microwave. Put on some topping (see Rice Cakes toppings) and you have a tasty treat. For a change use a sweet potato.

Omelettes (200 kcal)

Omelettes are nice and filling. A 4 egg omelette adds up to 320 kcal and then you can put in 80 kcal of low calorie filling like mushrooms or spinach. Serves 2. Eat it slowly.

Soups

A large bowl (or even better, 2 bowls) of soup can be nourishing and fill you up at the same time. The basic starter here is microwaved chopped onion and garlic which you can use as a basis for lots of soups. Soups can be made ahead of time and put in a flask to take to work for lunch or eaten for your evening meal. Here are a few ideas which you can modify according to how creative you're feeling:

My Notes

Roasted Red Pepper Soup (355 kcal)

1 onion and some garlic = 70 kcal

3 red peppers = 90 kcal

2 teaspoons olive oil = 80 kcal

2 pints (about 1 liter) water

1 tablespoon fennel seeds = 5 kcal

14oz (400g) can of chopped

tomatoes = 90 kcal

salt and pepper

small bunch of fresh basil

Method

Chop up the onion and garlic. Microwave on full with a little water for around 5 mins or until the onions are soft. Put in a big pan on a medium heat.

Preheat oven to 180^0C (356^0F).

Cut peppers into strips, removing seeds and roast with oil in oven for 40 mins.

Put all ingredients (except basil) into pan, bring to boil and simmer for 20 mins.

Liquidize soup and return to pan to warm through. Serve in bowls garnished with roughly chopped basil.

Butternut Squash Soup (220 kcal)

1 onion and some garlic = 70 kcal
1 14oz (400g) butternut squash = 150 kcal
2 pints (about 1 liter) water
salt and pepper

Method
Chop up the onion and garlic. Microwave on full with a little water for around 5 mins or until the onions are soft. Put in a big pan on a medium heat.
Remove seeds from the butternut squash and chop up.
Put everything into pan, bring to boil then simmer for 30 mins. Liquidize, return to pan, heat up, and voila! Lots of soup for little calories and you don't even have to share this one!

Zucchini (Courgette) and Mint Soup

(145 kcal)

1 onion and some garlic = 70 kcal

3 large zucchinis = 75 kcal

1 pint (about 2 liters) water

salt and pepper

5 sprigs of mint

Method

Chop up the onion and garlic. Microwave on full with a little water for around 5 mins or until the onions are soft. Put in a big pan on a medium heat.

Add chopped zucchinis, water and mint.

Season with salt and pepper.

Bring to boil, simmer for 30 mins.

Blend soup and there you go – lots of soup for hardly any calories.

My Notes

Iris's Pea Soup (300 kcal)

With thanks to Clive's mum for this one – this makes easily enough for 2.

7oz (200g) frozen peas = 130 kcal
1 liter (about 2 pints) water
2 onions and some garlic = 140 kcal
chopped mint or parsley
2 tablespoons low fat yoghurt = 30 kcal
salt and pepper

Method

Finely chop the onions and garlic. Microwave on full with a little water for around 5 mins or until the onions are soft. Put in a big pan on a medium heat.

Add the frozen peas and water, bring to boil and simmer for 10 mins.

Add herbs, salt and pepper.

Blend soup in blender and return to pan.

Off the heat, add the yoghurt and stir in.

Ready to serve!

Carrot Soup (190 kcal)

Carrot soup is a winner and there are lots of variations on this theme.

1 onion and some garlic = 70 kcal

3 large carrots = 120 kcal

1 pint (about 2 liters) water

salt and pepper

Method

Chop up the onion and garlic. Microwave on full with a little water for around 5 mins or until the onions are soft. Put in a big pan on a medium heat.

Peel and grate carrots.

Add ingredients to pan then simmer for 30 mins then blend and there you go.

And then you can add the following:

My Notes

Carrot and Orange Soup - Add juice of one large orange (extra 40 kcal)

Carrot and Herb Soup - Just add your favorite herb like tarragon or cilantro (coriander) and you've created a new soup!

Carrot and Ginger Soup - Add 1 teaspoon of ginger powder (or 1 tablespoon of grated ginger) at the simmering stage (almost no extra calories).

My Notes

Evening Meals

These recipes serve 2 and work out at a maximum of 400 kcal for the whole thing. You should get 2 bowls of food each which is psychologically very satisfying.

Top tip – there's no need to use oil for the base of these dishes! Especially when you think that one teaspoon of oil is 40 kcal! So we've microwaved everything where necessary.

Spicy Chili (325 kcal)

10oz (300g) mushrooms = 40 kcal
half tin of kidney beans = 125 kcal
2 medium onions = 60 kcal
3 garlic cloves = 10 kcal
14oz (400g) tin chopped tomatoes = 90 kcal
1oz (30ml) water
1 teaspoon chili powder, half teaspoon of ground cumin,

ground cilantro (coriander), turmeric, black pepper, salt to taste.

Method

Finely chop the onions and garlic. Microwave on full with a little water for around 5 mins or until the onions are soft. Put in a big pan on a medium heat.

Add the mushrooms and stir occasionally for a further 5 mins (keep lid on)

Add kidney beans and stir.

Add chopped tomatoes and water.

Add herbs and spices.

Bring to boil and simmer with lid on for 1 hour, stirring occasionally.

My Notes

Super Quantity Veg Curry (320 kcal)

10oz (300g) mushrooms = 40 kcal

7oz (200g) small cauliflower florets = 70 kcal

2 medium onions = 60 kcal

3 garlic cloves = 10 kcal

2 medium carrots = 50 kcal

14oz (400g) tin chopped tomatoes = 90 kcal

1oz (30ml) water

1 teaspoon curry powder, half teaspoon of ground cumin,

ground cilantro (coriander), turmeric, black pepper, salt to taste.

Method

Finely chop the onions and garlic. Microwave on full with a little water for around 5 mins or until the onions are soft. Put in a big pan on a medium heat.

Peel and coarsely grate the carrots.

Add the mushrooms and stir occasionally for a further 5 mins (keep lid on)

Add the carrots, cauliflower and stir.

Add herbs and spices, chopped tomatoes and water.

Bring to boil and simmer with lid on for 1 hour, stirring occasionally.

Eat and enjoy!

There are lots of variations on the above basic curry recipe. For example:

Spinach and Chickpea Curry: in the basic curry replace the tomatoes by a bag of spinach = 30 kcal and half a tin of chickpeas = 125 kcal.

Cauliflower and Potato Curry: in the basic curry replace the tomatoes and carrots by 9oz (250g) of potatoes = 190 kcal.

My Notes

Zucchini (Courgette) and Bean Curry

(330 kcal)

5oz (150g) onion = 50 kcal

2 cloves garlic = 10 kcal

7oz (200g) mushrooms = 30 kcal

9oz (250g) zucchini (courgette) = 50 kcal

small tin haricot beans = 170 kcal

3oz (100ml) water

handful of cabbage = 20 kcal

1 teaspoon each of garam masala, turmeric, curry powder, ground cumin, salt and pepper

chopped fresh cilantro (coriander) to taste.

Method

Finely chop the onions and garlic. Microwave on full with a little water for around 5 mins or until the onions are soft. Put in a big pan on a medium heat.

Add chopped mushrooms, cover and cook for 5 mins.

In the meantime, coarsely grate the zucchini (courgette) and add to the pan, together with the haricot beans. Add the water and simmer for 5 mins.

Chop the cabbage finely and add to the pan. Add the herbs and spices, cover the pan and cook for 30 mins.

My Notes

Mushroom and Potato Stroganoff

(350 kcal)

7oz (200g) onions, 2 cloves garlic = 70 kcal

7oz (200g) mushrooms = 30 kcal

9oz (250g) new potatoes = 190 kcal

1.5oz (50ml) water

1.5oz (50ml) pot low fat yoghurt or crème fraiche = 60 kcal

salt, pepper and fresh tarragon if you fancy it

Method

Finely chop the onions and garlic. Microwave on full with a little water for around 5 mins or until the onions are soft. Put in a big pan on a medium heat.

Add to pan chopped mushrooms and water, cook down a bit.

In the meantime, dice the potatoes into small cubes and microwave for 5 mins with a bit of water.

Add the potatoes to the pan and cook everything together for about 10 mins making sure that the mix is not too watery.
Season to taste and add the yoghurt.

Mushrooms on Toast (360 kcal)

4 slices of medium sized wholemeal bread = 260 kcal

10oz (300g) mushrooms = 40 kcal

1.5oz (50ml) pot low fat yoghurt or crème fraiche = 60 kcal

salt and pepper

Method

Finely chop and microwave the mushrooms for about 3 mins and then drain off any water that has accumulated.

Meanwhile, toast your bread.

Mix in the tub of yoghurt with your mushrooms and then pour on the toast. Eat. Yum.

Fish/Prawn Curry (300 kcals)

Prawns are pretty low in calories as are white fish.

5oz (150g) prawns = 100 kcal *or* small piece of white fish = 100 kcal
10oz (300g) mushrooms = 40 kcal
2 medium onions = 60 kcal
3 garlic cloves = 10 kcal
14oz (400g) tin chopped tomatoes = 90 kcal
1oz (30ml) water
1 teaspoon curry powder, half teaspoon of ground cumin,
ground cilantro (coriander), turmeric, black pepper, salt to taste.

Method

Finely chop the onions and garlic. Microwave on full with a little water for around 5 mins or until the onions are soft. Put in a big pan on a medium heat.

Add the mushrooms and stir occasionally for a further 5 mins (keep lid on)
Add the prawns or fish.
Add herbs and spices, chopped tomatoes and the water.
Bring to boil and simmer with lid on for 1 hour, stirring occasionally.
Eat and enjoy!

It's easy to change this to become a fish/prawn bouillabaisse by adding a few potatoes and tomatoes and taking out the curry ingredients!

My Notes

Sweet Potato Casserole (355 kcal)

7oz (200g) sweet potato = 165kcal

14oz (400g) tin chopped tomatoes = 90 kcal

1 onion and some garlic = 70 kcal

7oz (200g) mushrooms = 30 kcal

salt and pepper

chopped fresh basil and teaspoon chili powder

Method

Heat the oven to 180°C (356°F).

Finely chop the onions and garlic. Microwave on full with a little water for around 5 mins or until the onions are soft. Put them into a casserole dish with the tomatoes, cubed sweet potatoes and chopped mushrooms. Add the seasoning and then bake the whole thing (lid on) for about 40 mins in the oven – irresistible.

Shazzie's Fish Stew (420 kcal)

6oz (180g) of frozen pollock or similar white fish = 180 kcal

7oz (200g) onion, 2 cloves garlic = 70 kcal

14oz (400g) tin tomatoes = 90 kcal

3.5oz (100g) new potatoes = 80 kcal

fresh basil and thyme to season along with salt and pepper

Method

Finely chop the onions and garlic. Microwave on full with a little water for around 5 mins or until the onions are soft. Put them in a pan together with the diced fish and tomatoes. Stir and simmer whilst you cube and microwave the potatoes for 5 mins or so. Add potatoes to the pan and simmer all together with seasoning (lid on pan) for 15 mins.

Stir-Fries

Stir-fries are a great way of getting lots of healthy veg in a tasty way. You need to stay away from ready-made sauces so just add a bit of soy/fish/oyster sauce to your finished stir-fry and you won't have too many calories.

Here's a basic stir-fry recipe. After reading through our book you should be ready to add and experiment with your favorite ingredients to make your own signature dish – do let us know about your inventions!

Chicken Stir-Fry (387 kcal)

10oz (300g) mushrooms = 40 kcal

2 medium onions = 60 kcal

3 garlic cloves = 10 kcal

7oz (200g) breast of chicken = 212 kcal

bag spinach = 15 kcal

1 teaspoon oil = 40 kcal

2 tablespoons soy sauce = 10 kcal

Method

Heat the oil in a wok on a fairly high heat. Add sliced onions and crushed garlic and stir-fry for 2 mins until they start to soften and gain some color.

Cut the chicken into thin strips and add to stir-fry for 3 mins then add the mushrooms and spinach and keep stirring for another few minutes. Everything should be nicely cooked and smelling great at this stage.

Add the soy sauce, stir through and there you go! Tasty stir fry.

You can vary this by using turkey or quorn instead of chicken and using different veggies too.

My Notes

Drinks

Water does not contain any calories and is a good way to fill up if your stomach is rumbling.

Cup of black tea or coffee = 1 kcal
Cup of tea with semi-skimmed (2%) milk and 1 teaspoon sugar = 26 kcal
Small glass (3oz, 100ml) of pure fruit juice = 100 kcal
Small glass (3oz, 100ml) of semi-skimmed (2%) milk = 50 kcal

My Notes

Freebies (Very Low Calorie Foods)

Cup of tea (black, green, any color you like) without milk or sugar

Glass of water

Zero coke (if you really must)

Stick of celery

Flavored teas

Black coffee – don't go mad or you'll be crawling on the ceiling

My Notes

Snacks

Yes, snacking is bad, blah, blah, blah. But you might have the odd few calories to use up and you might want to combine some snacks to make one meal so why not have a (small calorie) ball? Here are some ideas that should be no more than 50 kcals:

10 olives (apparently they are good for the liver although maybe not if you combine them with gin and tonic)

7 almonds

1 Jaffa Cake (but could you stop at one?)

1 small apple

miso soup in powder sachets

2 celery sticks stuffed with cottage cheese (yuk, Clive)

3 squares of good quality chocolate – get the high cocoa content

15 grapes

half a melon

3 dried apricots

13 cherries

2 satsumas

10 chocolate coated raisins

2 slices of mango

a small jar of cocktail gherkins (you've got to be kidding me, Clive)

2 kiwi fruits

16 strawberries

1 medium peach

1 rice cake with a smidge of peanut butter

My Notes

Calorie Counter

Here are some approximate calorie figures for common 'fasting' foods. We haven't included foods with a high calorific content (like chocolate and meat pies) because there's no point as you wouldn't be able to eat much of them on your 'fasting' days (although you can eat them on your 'feasting' days of course).

Unless given in a more convenient way, the following figures show the calorie content of common foods by weight. You're going to need kitchen scales and a calculator which is a bit tedious but you will soon remember the calorific values for your favorite recipes. Most foods have their calorific values printed on their packaging so always check.

Vegetables and Salads (approximate kcals, per 100g / per oz)

Broccoli 33/9
Cabbage 26/7

Carrots 35/10

Cauliflower 34/10

Cucumber 10/3

Lettuce, and other salad leaves 15/4

Mushroom 13/4

Onions 36/10

Peas 83/24

Potatoes 75/21

Tomatoes 17/5

Rocket 15/4

Watercress 15/4

Zucchinis (Courgettes) 18/5

Beans and Pulses (approximate kcals, per 100g / per oz)

Chickpeas, canned 115/33

Kidney Beans, canned 100/28

(remember to check calorific values printed on the tins)

Fish and Seafood (approximate kcals, per 100g / per oz)

Haddock, cod, pollock uncooked 80/23

Prawns 99/28

Trout, grilled 135/38

Tuna in brine 99/28

Tuna in oil 189/54

Mackerel, uncooked 170/48

Meat (approximate kcals, per 100g / per oz)

Chicken fillet, uncooked 106/30

Turkey, uncooked 105/30

Ham, sliced 100/28

Chorizo, small slice 15/4 (a little of this goes a long way for flavor)

Dairy, Fats and Oils (approximate kcals, per 100g / per oz)

Milk, whole 66/19

Milk, semi-skimmed (2%) 50/14

Milk, skimmed (1%) 33/9

Fromage frais, very low fat 58/16

Low fat yoghurt, plain 56/16

Lard 900/255 (just joking, don't do it!)

Eggs, medium 80/23

Reduced fat Greek yoghurt 80/23

Cereals and Preserves

Sugar, 1 teaspoon 16

Honey, 1 teaspoon 25

Rice cake 25

Crispbread 25

Small packet of oat biscuits 100

Oats, 1.5oz (40g) serving 150

My Notes

Fruit (approximate kcals, per 100g / per oz)

Apple 50/14

Avocado 190/54

Banana 95/27

Grapefruit 30/9

Orange 37/10

Peach 33/9

Pear 40/11

Melon 28/8

Strawberries 27/8

Rhubarb 10/3 (this is your friend)

My Notes

Add Your Favorites Here

Tips

The problem with diets is that they can be hard to stick to. In order to keep to this diet and get the health benefits we have tried to make it as easy as possible to follow. Here's what we do:

- Write the number of kcal on cans and packets of your 'fasting' foods to avoid having to consult the Calorie Counter all the time. Stick labels on your fridge door with the calorific values of your favorite 'fasting' foods on.
- Eat slowly with a small spoon to make your 'fasting' food last longer.
- Eat your 'fasting' food from a small bowl and have seconds.
- Have a glass of water with your meal as this will fill you up.
- Trade calories to get something you like. For example, Clive used to start the day with calorie-free black tea

which he hated. He now has his usual tea with milk and sugar (26 kcal) and a bit less porridge but is happier.
- Get a friend or partner to do the diet with you that way you can encourage each other.

Add Your Tips Here

Results

After 12 weeks on the Feast and Fast Diet Clive's 'bad' (LDL) cholesterol went down by 20% and both Mags (48 years old, 5ft (1.52m)) and Clive (53 years old, 5ft 10in (1.8m)) experienced weight losses of approximately 1lb (0.5kg) per week. Our figures were:

Clive's cholesterol readings (mmol/L)			
	Total	HDL	LDL
Before	7.0	1.1	5.0
After	6.2	1.0	4.0

Our weights	
	Mags	Clive
Before	112lb (51kg)	163lb (74kg)
After	99lb (45kg)	154lb, (70kg)

We have both lost our middle-aged spread and friends say that we look healthier. We certainly feel healthier. It seems that Clive's weight has stabilized but Mags is continuing to lose weight so she may have to modify her diet before she wastes away! We haven't had much of a problem incorporating the diet in to our lives but occasionally, where it has been impossible to have a 'fasting' evening meal, we have fasted completely until the following 'feasting' evening meal to make up for it.

We both experienced hunger pangs at around 9pm on 'fasting' days for the first couple of weeks but these reduced over time. One massive change is that for years Mags used to have a complete melt-down whenever she got hungry: this no longer happens (Clive is very pleased). It seems that something has changed in her response to hunger. Another unexpected benefit is that we both appreciate food more and no longer take it for granted.

The next step for Clive is to increase his good (HDL) cholesterol by eating more oily fish on 'feasting' days.

We aim to continue this diet indefinitely because of the many reported health benefits.

Good luck with your Feast and Fast adventure!

Mags and Clive, February 2013.

Printed in Great Britain
by Amazon